THE ART OF PHLEBOTOMY

THE ART OF PHLEBOTOMY

PROCEDURES MANUAL

GUIDE/ SKILLS HANDBOOK

RENEE BLACKMON

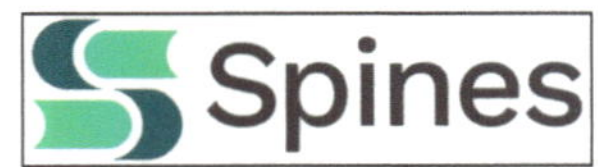

CONTENTS

This book is written with the intent to help healthcare workers and the public with the facts, information, and skills acquired by Phlebotomy Training Center of Ohio, through experience and education.

This book will also help with understanding the definition of phlebotomy, the equipment a phlebotomist uses, what areas to avoid, policies and procedures, dermal puncture, common tubes, the order of draw, and more to aid in future and past prospects in the healthcare field.

This book will enhance knowledge and skills for many who are in healthcare and those who are thinking of becoming a healthcare phlebotomist. The book will also support the development of more confidence and professionalism as you embark upon a phlebotomy position. Additionally, your strategies will become uplifted as you master the skill. Your technique will be your own.

This book will show you how to master the challenging situations a phlebotomist encounters day by day and to soothe the apprehensiveness that a patient may have with empathy and therapeutic techniques. Sit back and learn the journey of the "Art of Phlebotomy."

According to Merriam-Webster.com (10/5/2024) Phlebotomy is a surgical opening of a vein; the drawing of blood (as by venipuncture) for transfusion, apheresis, diagnostic testing, or experimental procedures," or "bloodletting."

The process of phlebotomy is the incision of a needle into a vein, from the arm, capillary, or foot (physician's order) to procure blood and provide results for a doctor's treatment of a patient.

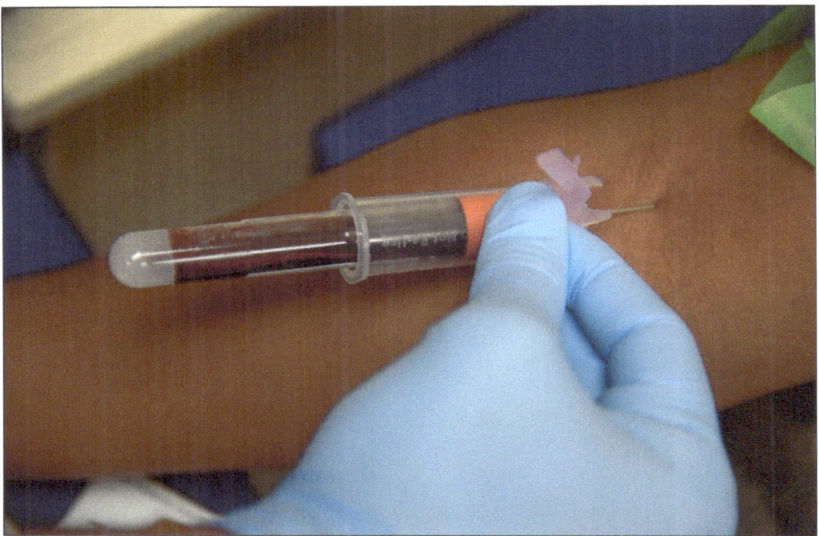

EQUIPMENT

What equipment is used for phlebotomy? During a phlebotomy procedure, there is special equipment that a phlebotomist must use, such as:

A tourniquet (elastic band) which is used to place around an adult or child's arm or(with a doctor's order) the foot , to stop the flow of blood, making it easy to fill vacutainer tubes.

Vacutainer tubes are used to receive blood when performing a venipuncture

Seventy percent isopropyl alcohol" is used to clean a site.

Needle (21-22G) to perform a venipuncture

Needle holder (hub) is used to hold the 21-22g needle in place

Gauze (2x2) is used to wipe away alcohol or blood and to apply pressure to site

"Gloves are worn: vinyl or Nitrile one set per patient

A bandage is used to place on the incision during postop

Sharps Container are used to deposit needles, needle units for safety

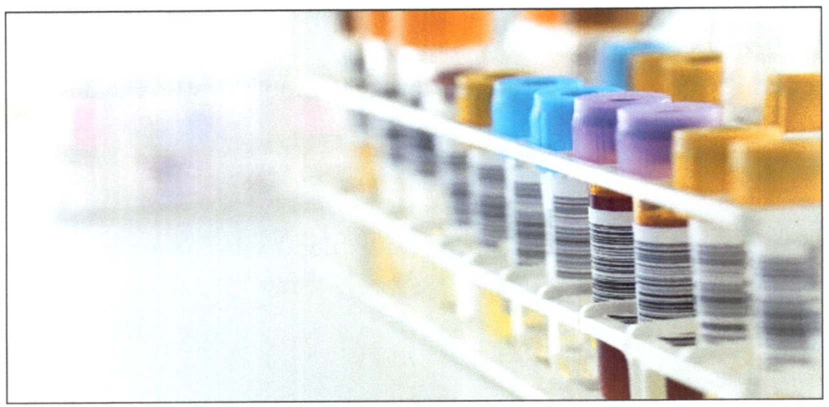

VENIPUNCTURE

One of the scariest things in life for most people is to have their blood drawn. Here are the steps to help with apprehensiveness:

1. Wash your hands.
2. Introduce yourself with your title, smile, and be warm/friendly)
3. Ask for two identifiers (Name/DOB) patient has to state their name/date of birth
4. Look at your requisition to compare (see nurse if it conflicts)
5. Explain to your patient why you are there in an easy to understandable manner
6. Assemble your equipment (in the correct order of draw; test)
7. Ask your patient (in a kind manner) which arm is the best to perform their draw
8. Ask them to roll their sleeves, make a fist and to keep arm extended throughout the draw
9. If the arm they choose is not suitable ask if you could try the other arm
10. Tie the tourniquet on the arm in a cris-cross manner so bunny ears will point at the top 2-4 in
11. Palpate (feel) for a vein
12. Use 70% Isopropyl to cleanse site/let dry 30 seconds
13. Anchor the vein
14. Keep the bevel up insert the 21-22g needle in the direction of the vein (swift/smooth).
15. Insert one vacutainer tube, place two fingers on the tips of the hub and using the thumb to push the tube upward to break the seal and receive blood

16. Remove the tourniquet by grabbing one of the bunny ears, let it drop (less than 1minute)

17. Remove the tube by using two fingers under the bottom of tube to cradle and the thumb to message the tube outward

18. Place tube down and invert once

19. Take your 2x2 and place it over the needle, pull out of the patients vein simultaneously click safety on needle and deposit it in sharps container and apply pressure to the site

20. Ask patient to hold pressure with the 2x2

21. You are to invert tube(s) 6-8 times ; label tube with patient name, dob, military time, date, and your initials

22. Post-op check your patient, place bandage on site

23. Place all tubes in a specimen bag

24. Wash your hands

25. Depart warmly from your patient

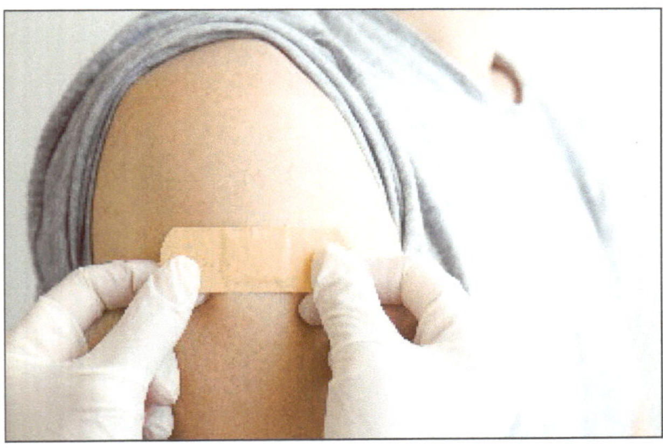

AREAS TO AVOID

There are certain areas that must be avoided during a venipuncture, due to infection, pain, hemolysis, specimen contamination, decreased blood flow, or injury to the patient. The areas include:

Mastectomy	Will cause infection; opposite side to procure blood
Fistula	Will cause infection/and injury from the surgery; opposite side will be sufficient to procure blood
Edema	Will cause contamination; draw opposite side
Scars	Will cause pain and decreased blow flow; hemolysis
Tatoo	Will cause contamination, less than a year
Wrist	Will cause contamination; this is arterial blood
IV	Will cause contamination; shut iv off 5 mins (nurse)
Foot	May cause infection (need a doctor's order) permission

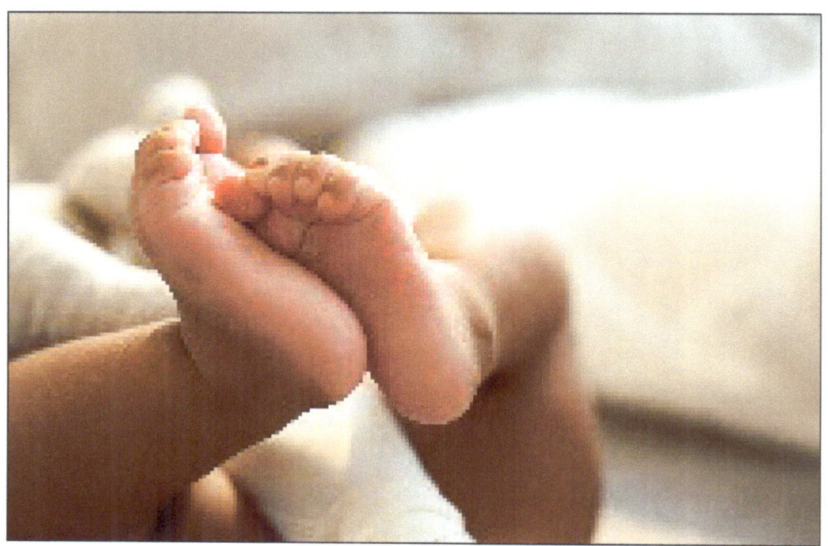

There are guidelines that The Center of Control and Prevention (CDC)regulates when it comes to breaking the chain of infection. The policies are all the same in most facilities.

Handwashing

1. Wet hands with warm, running water
2. Apply antibacterial soap on both hands
3. Rub both hands together to bring a lather and to loosen debris.
4. Completely clean hands for 20 seconds;(sing Happy birthday song) and be sure to wash

All fingers, under nails, under wedding band/ring, thumb, and wrist.

1. Rinse one hand at a time in a downward motion to prevent water splashes and recontamination.
2. Get a paper towel to dry your hands
3. Get a paper towel off the faucet.

Note: Alcohol-based sanitizer is good to use when hands are not visibly soiled.

1. Apply sanitizer in the palm of your hand. Rub your hands together until the agent has dissolved.

Note: Sanitizers are not intended to replace antibacterial soap and water.

Note: Gloves are to be worn after each patient.

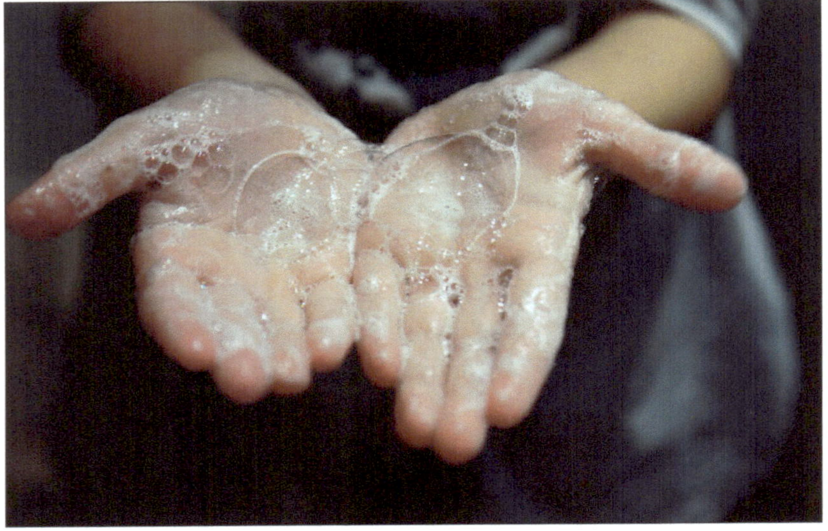

When drawing blood from a patient, there could be many setbacks. We will list a few and learn.

Hemoconcentration
Cause

1.	Long-term iv-therapy	Decrease IV time
2.	Probing	Stick once swift and smooth
3.	Prolonged Tourniquet	Less than a minute

Hemolysis
Cause (Performance Errors)

1.	Prolong Tourniquet	Less than a minute
2.	Improper Inversion	Do not shake; gently rock tube
3.	Improper Centrifugation	Centrifuge tubes for appropriate time

Failure to obtain blood
Cause

1.	Bevel against wall of vein	Pull needle back; anchor, change tube
2.	Deep Insertion	Pull needle back; stay inside the vein
3.	Needles	Use 21-22g; winged infusion
4.	Dehydration	hydrate for better blood flow
5.	Technique	Stay in alignment of the vein direction

Hematomas
Cause

1.	Inadequate Pressure	Place full pressure on draw site(2x2)
2.	Large Needle	Use appropriate size needle
3.	Partial Needle Placement	Place needle far enough in vein
4.	Injury	Do not place needle past the vein

Note:

If a hematoma occurs discontinue the venipuncture, by removing the tourniquet and needle. Apply pressure to the site and offer a cold compress to reduce the swelling. And consult your supervisor on your policies.

DERMAL PUNCTURE

When performing a dermal puncture, there are several things to consider:

FINGER STICK

1. After introductions, handwashing and getting two identifiers from the patient (name/DOB)
2. Ask Patient which is his/her dominant hand; and use the non-dominant hand
3. Explain to the patient that you need to use the middle or ring finger
4. Place your gloves on; begin to wipe the middle or ring finger with 70% isopropyl alcohol
5. Using a lancet, puncture the ring or middle finger; (sides)then wipe the first blood
6. Squeeze finger until blood appears; Using a capillary tube place it on the ball of blood; repeat the method until the capillary tube is filled; place tube in a clay tray.

HEEL STICK

1. Wash Hands
2. Identify the infant by looking at the requisition, armband and/or ankle band
3. Gather equipment
4. Position infant on his back
5. Select a site using the medial and lateral areas of the sides of the foot(Plantar)
6. Grasp the infant's foot with your hand; so that stability is achieved
7. Wipe the side id the heel with 70% isopropyl alcohol
8. Puncture the heel (medial) and (lateral) with a lancet to achieve a ball of blood
9. Wipe the first blood and alcohol with a 2x2
10. Start to obtain blood in a capillary tube and /or screening card or micro container until full
11. Once the blood has been achieved, apply pressure until bleeding stops , then bandage the site.
12. Label the necessary tubes and forms; post-op for your patient
13. Remove gloves
14. Wash hands

Note:

Do Not puncture the posterior aspect of the infant's heel. Dermal puncture is the method chosen for collecting blood from infants and
Children younger than 2 years old; and adults with inaccessible or fragile veins.

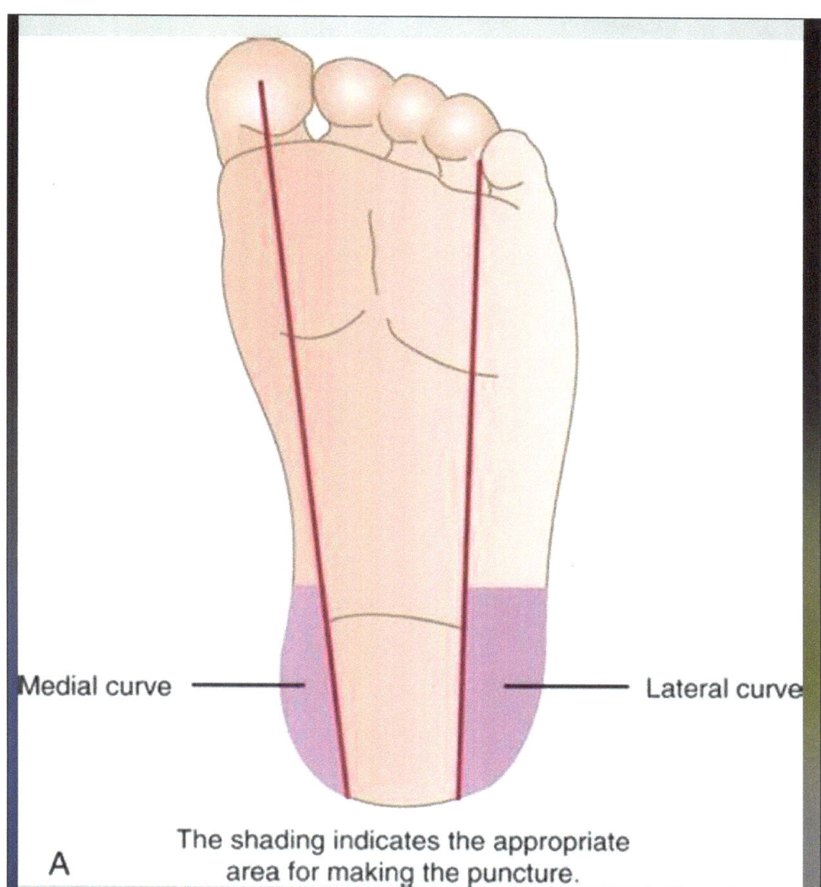

The shading indicates the appropriate area for making the puncture.

A

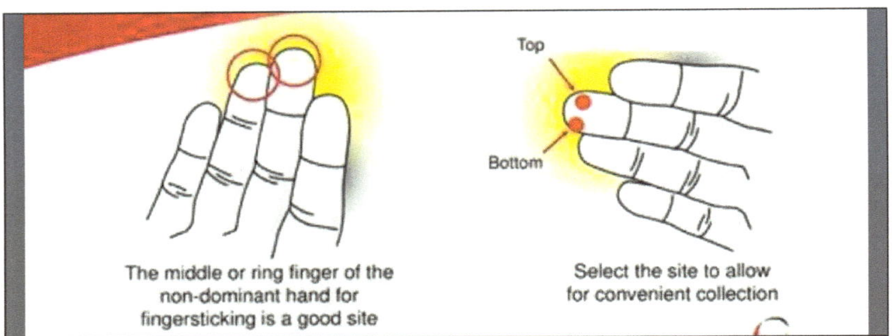

The middle or ring finger of the
non-dominant hand for
fingersticking is a good site

Select the site to allow
for convenient collection

Note: Avoid scarred areas

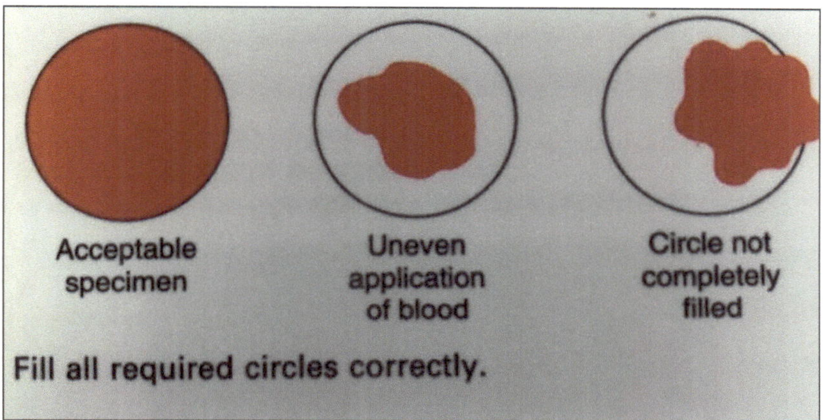

Note: Avoid touching blood on the filtered paper

Note: Uneven and incomplete applications will result in a Rejected and unprocessed status

SPECIAL COLLECTIONS

When collecting blood specimens from a patient, there are certain aspects you will have to consider that relies greatly on the results. There are special ways to transport, collect and handle some specimens once drawn. Here are a few examples:

<table>
<tr><td>

ICE
Ammonia
Latic Acid – no tourniquet
pH
PHT

</td><td>

OGTT
REQUIRES 4 DRAWS
baseline; every hour up to 4

</td></tr>
<tr><td>

LIGHT PROTECTION
Bilirubin

B12
Porphyrins

</td><td>

SST
PERMITS A 15-minute wait time
before spun
must clot first.

</td></tr>
<tr><td>

FILLED
ESR (2/3)
PT (capacity)

D-Dimer
Fibringin

</td><td>

Blood Cultures
sterile procedure; requires 2 draws
anaerobic/aerobic; must use a
butterfly needle.

</td></tr>
<tr><td>

REFRIGERATE
24 HOUR URINE
CANCER ANTIGEN
ANTISTREPTOLSIN

</td><td>

PT/PTT/INR
Must be filled; A red top tube
is required to use a waste tube

</td></tr>
</table>

COMMONLY USED TUBES

1. Serum Separator Tube
2. Lavender Top Tube
3. Green Top Tube
4. Pink Top Tube
5. Red Top Tube
6. Gray Top Tube
7. Gold Top Tube
8. Blue Top Tube

COMMON ABBREVIATIONS

1	CBC	Complete Blood Count
2	BMP	Basic Metabolic Panel
3	CMP	Comprehensive Metabolic Panel
4	TSH	Thyroid Stimulating Hormone
5	PT	Prothrombin Time
6	OGTT	Oral Glucose Tolerance Testing
7	ESR	Estimate Sedimentation Rate
8	WSR	Western Sedimentation Rate
9	WBC	White Blood Count
10	RBC	Red Blood Count
11	BCX	Blood Culture
12	Amm	Ammonia
13	BAT	Blood Alcohol Test
14	Hct	Hemacrit
15	Hgb	Hemoglobin
16	K	Potassium
17	PSA	Prostate-specific antigen
18	LI	Lithium
19	Mg	Magnesium
20	Billi	Bilirubin

<h1 style="text-align:center">ORDER OF DRAW</h1>

When collecting blood specimen, it is very important to keep the sequence of the order because following the order helps prevent cross-contamination, leading to more accurate patient test results. There are over 25 or more tubes. In this quick reference book, I can provide you with a few.

1.	BCX	8 to 10x	invert
2.	Light Blue	3 to 4x	invert
3.	Red	5 to 8x	invert
4.	SST	5 to 8x	invert
5.	Green	5 to 8x	invert
6.	Lavender	8 to 10x	invert
7.	Gray	8 to 10x	invert

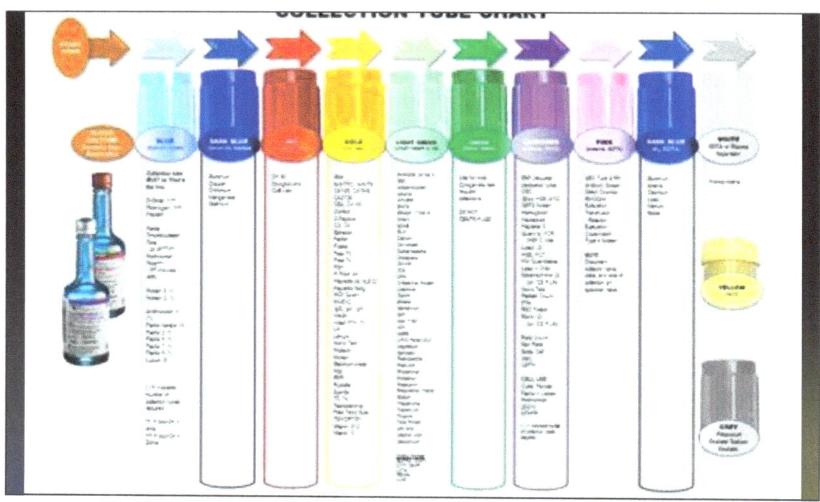

VOCABULARY

Hematoma	a bruise from a needle stick; prolonged tourniquet application
Syncope:	loss of consciousness; fainting
Hemolyze:	destruction of a red blood cell
Hemoconcentration	plasma; high amount
Centrifuge	a machine used to spin blood tubes; separate cells
Tourniquet	an elastic band used to stop blow flow
Capillary tube	an elongated glass tube used during a dermal puncture
PPE	Personal Protective Equipment; used for isolation
Fomite	an inanimate object
Neonate	infant
Wing infusion	23 g butterfly needle
Lancet	a small device with a needle encased, used for heel or finger stick
2x2	a white gauge used to clean and apply pressure
Hub	is also called needle holder; hold needle in place
RBC	red blood cell
WBC	white blood cell
Anchor	prevent movement; steady
Bevel	the opening of a slope
Requisition	work order; official order laying out claim to be performed
CDC	Centers for Disease Control and Prevention

LABS

TEST	COLLECTION TUBE	DEPARTMENT
BMP	SST	CHEMISTRY
CBC	LAVENDER	HEMATOLOGY
OGTT	GRAY	SPECIAL CHEMISTRY
CM	PINK	BLOOD BANK
PT	BLUE	COAGULATION
BCX	YELLOW	MICROBIOLOGY
IgM	RED	IMMUOLOGY

<h1 style="text-align:center">ACTIVITIES and GAMES</h1>

<h2 style="text-align:center">SCRAMBLE</h2>

To start, add a few test names on your tubes. For example, "BMP" should go in the SST in the correct order of draw. Your tubes should line up as in the example above. Now, with the second player of the game, ask them to call out the test, and you will move the tube you think is the right tube forward, keeping the tubes straight and in order. Once the test has been called out, the order should still fall in the correct order, no matter what!

You can play this game alone or with others. The purpose of this game is to keep the correct order, prevent contamination, avoid false readings—and to have fun!

<h2 style="text-align:center">MEMORY</h2>

Place your tubes in the correct order of draw. Then label them numerically. Place test labs on the label of the tubes. Now point at each tube and try to remember which lab to take them to. Do the same process with the labs now! Have fun! This game will enhance your memory for phlebotomy.

<h2 style="text-align:center">PHLEBOTOMY JEOPARDY</h2>

On a board or separate sheet of paper, write down categories (lab, tube, test, scenario)

Under the category list dollar amount (100,200 etc). List questions under your tabs, split up in groups take turns answering the phlebotomy questions until all categories have been played. This game is fun. And will increase your knowledge in phlebotomy.

PHLEBOTOMY SCRIPT (VENIPUNTURE)

Hello my name is________________
And I will be your phlebotomist.

Can you tell me your first and last name,
    with your date of birth?

Are you fasting?

Are you taking any aspirin or blood
    thinners?

Which arm is the best?

If I don't feel anything, may I look to find a
    vein in your other arm?

Thank you!

Note: Say this repeatedly until you have
    mastered it!

PHLEBOTOMY SCRIPT (FINGER STICK)

Hello my name is __________

I will be your phlebotomist.

Can you state your first and last name, with your date of birth?

Which is your dominant hand?

Great!

I will be using your non-dominant hand for your fingerstick.

And it involves your ring or middle finger.

Note: Rehearse until you have mastered it!

Thank you!

ACTIVITY

1. What tubes require ice?
2. What tubes should be protected by light?
3. What is a fomite?
4. Define Hemoconcentration
5. Put tubes in correct sequence.
6. What is meant by "syncope
7. Which tubes required to be filled to capacity?
8. How many draws do a OGTT require?
9. What is Phlebotomy?
10. How much alcohol is required to cleanse a site?

PHLEBOTOMY REQUISITION EXAMPLE

Community Physician   ♔ KAISER PERMANENTE. LABORATORY REQUISITION

UPIN / NPI# _______________________

Provider Name:

ADDRESS: ______________________________

PHONE NUMBER: _______________________

SECURE FAX NUMBER: ___________________

Required
ICD 9 DIAGNOSIS CODE(s):

**Medicare does not generally cover routine screening tests.

FILL IN ALL INFORMATION
- ❏ MALE
- ❏ FEMALE   DATE OF BIRTH: __________

PATIENT NAME: LAST   FIRST

iKAISER MEDICAL RECORD #

- ❏ NON- FASTING   ❏ STAT   ❏ ASAP
- ❏ FASTING HOURS ____   ❏ ROUTINE

Providers FAX this signed and dated form to: 303-404-4030

URINALYSIS
- ❏ 81003 UA reflex MICRO if positive- 81002
- ❏ 87088 URNC/CULTURE (reflexed as indicated)

HEMATOLOGY
- ❏ 85025 CBC/AUTO DIFF(man diff reflexed if meets criteria)
- ❏ 85652 ESR - SED RATE
- ❏ 85014/85018 Hemoglobin & Hematocrit
- ❏ 85046 RETICULOCYTE

COAGULATION
- ❏ 85610 PT PROTIME / INR
- ❏ 85730 PTT APTT

CHEMISTRY PROFILES
- ❏ 80048 **BMP** Chem 7 (LYTES,BUN,CREAT,GLU,CA)
- ❏ 80053 **CMP** Comp Metabolic Prof (BMP,HFP,TP)
- ❏ 80061 **FLIPP FASTING** (CHOL,TGL,HDL,LDL)
- ❏ 83550 / 83540 **IRPF** Iron Panel (FE,IBC,TIBC,TRANS SAT)
- ❏ 80076 **HFP** Hepatic Function Panel (ALB,AST,ALT,ALKP,TBIL/DBIL)
- ❏ 80051 **LYTES** (NA,K,CL,CO2)
- ❏ 80069 **RFP** (LYTES,BUN,CR,GLU,CA,ALB,PHOS)
- ❏ 84443 **THYP** FT4 reflexed if TSH abnormal FT3 reflexed if TSH low and FT4 norm

CHEMISTRY SINGLE TESTS
- ❏ 84460 ALT (SGPT)
- ❏ 82150 AMYLASE
- ❏ 84450 AST (SGOT)
- ❏ 82247 BILIRUBIN, TOTAL- ADULT
- ❏ 84520 BUN
- ❏ 82310 CALCIUM
- ❏ 82550 CPK
- ❏ 82565 CREATININE
- ❏ 82728 FERRITIN
- ❏ 82746 FOLATE   R
- ❏ 82947 GLUCOSE, ___ HRS PP
- ❏ 83036 HEMOGLOBIN A1C   LAV
- ❏ 84132 POTASSIUM
- ❏ 83690 LIPASE

- ❏ 83735 MAGNESIUM
- ❏ 84100 PHOSPHORUS
- ❏ 83970/82310/82565/84100 PTHINT INTACT PTH-Fasting preferred   SST & LAV
- ❏ 82043 / 82570 RMA   RAND URINE PROT/CREAT RATIO
- ❏ 84295 SODIUM
- ❏ 84443 TSH
- ❏ 84550 URIC ACID
- ❏ 82607 VITAMIN B12
- ❏ 82746/82607 VITAMIN B12/FOLATE

THERAPEUTIC DRUGS
DATE AND TIME OF LAST DOSE:

- ❏ 80162 DIGOXIN
- ❏ 80185 DILANTIN   R
- ❏ 80170 GENTAMYCIN   ❏ PEAK ❏ TROUGH
- ❏ 80178 LITHIUM
- ❏ 80156 TEGRETOL (CARBAMAZEPINE)
- ❏ 80164 VALPROIC ACID (DEPAKOTE)
- ❏ 80202 VANCOMYCIN   ❏ PEAK ❏ TROUGH

SPECIAL CHEMISTRY
- ❏ 86592 RPR SYPHLIS SCREEN
- ❏ 84165 SPEP SERUM PROT ELECTROPHORESIS
- ❏ 86706 HEPATITIS B SURFACE AB

OTHER TESTING
- ❏ GLUCOSE TOLERANCE (OB)
  - ❏ 82950 1 HOUR
  - ❏ 82947 (X2) 2 HOUR POST MEAL
  - ❏ 82947 (X4) 3 HOUR TOLERANCE
- ❏ 84703 SERUM PREG
- ❏ 81025 URINE PREG
- ❏ 84702 BETA HCG QUANT
- ❏ 82670 ESTRADIAL
- ❏ 84144 PROGESTERONE
- ❏ 83001 (+ 83002) LH/FSH

24 HOUR URINE TESTS
- ❏ 82575 CRCL   CREAT CLEARANCE W/ SERUM
- ❏ 82340 UCA   CALCIUM
- ❏ 84166 UPEP   URINE PROTEIN ELECTROPHORESIS
- ❏ 84156 UPROT TOTAL URINE PROTEIN

24 hour urine containers can be picked up at any Kaiser Permanente laboratory location.

No appointments necessary for routine laboratory testing at any Kaiser Permanente lab facility

No specimens will be accepted at any Kaiser Permanente facility

To Order Any Other Test.

Provider must call: 303-743-5330

The tests on this requisition have been approved by the attending physician.

____
Provider signature   Date

DRAW SITE ______ # OF STICKS ______   UNABLE TO DRAW ______   Physician notified? YES   NO

SST________ LAVENDER________ RED________ BLUE________ GREEN________ GRAY________ URINE________ STOOL________ SWAB________

COMMENTS: LABORATORY LOCATION   RECEIVED BY

Phlebotomy Quiz Example

Name: ____   Date: ________

phlebotomy quiz

1. What is osteoporosis?	A. red blood cells
2. ABG	B. bloodtyping
3. ABO	C. bleeding time
4. ACD	D. arterial blood gases
5. bc or b/c	E. magnesium
6. BT	F. hematocrit
7. Ca	G. blood culture
8. CHOL	H. calcium
9. ETOH	I. acid citrate dextrose
10. Fe	J. iron
11. Hct	K. electrolytes
12. Lytes	L. ethanol
13. Mg++	M. will make the bone weak.
14. RBC	N. cholesterol

RESOURCES AND REFERENCES

USEFUL WEBSITES

- Center for Disease Control and Prevention: www.cdc.gov/index
- Center for Phlebotomy Education; www.orderofdraw.
- Complications of Phlebotomy: www.needle.tube/resource-8/common-risk-complication
- Phlebotomy Training Center of Ohio: www.phlebotomytraining centerohio.com

REFERENCE

American Merriam Dictionary. (2024). "What is Phlebotomy?"
Centers for Disease Control and Prevention. (2024). "Preventing Infection in Hand-washing and Safety." CDC.
CLSI. (2024). "Procedures of handling test tubes and Processing Blood Clinical and Laboratory Institute, Wayne, PA 2012.